This Essential Oils Journal Belongs To:

_____

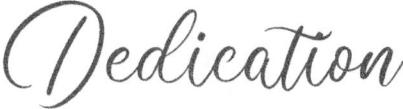

This Essential Oil Journal is dedicated to individuals looking for the natural healing benefits of aromatherapy and essential oils.

You are my inspiration for producing this book and I'm honored to be a part of your wellness and self care through the power of essential oils.

How to Use this Book

This Essential Oil Journal will help you organize your oils and recipes and provide you with basic and seasonal recipes. This easy to use book will provide you with unique recipes, as well as worksheets to test out blends and much more.

Here are examples for tracking your oils and blends, recipes, plus inventory lists.

1. My favorite Oils - Fill out these pages for your favorite blends for energy, calming, sleep, wellness, etc.

2. Essential Oil Recipes - Record your favorite recipes.

3. Testing Out Blends - Fill out name, purpose, ingredients and notes.

4. My Oil Ratings - Write purpose of oil, name of oil and your rating.

5. My Favorite Blends - Record your favorite blends.

6. Essential Oil Wish List - Fill out your oil wish list.

7. Blends - A variety of blends for lavender, wellness, happiness, seasonal and more.

8. Essential Oil Inventory - Fill out your inventory list.

Essential Oil Inventory

NAME	USED FOR	DATE OPENED	FAVORITE?

Essential Oil Wish List

NAME	USED FOR	PRICE	KID SAFE?

My Favorite Oils

ENERGY

CALMING

SLEEP

FOCUS/CLARITY

WELLNESS

ROMANCE

ANXIETY

JOYFUL

Testing Out Blends

NAME:

INGREDIENTS:

PURPOSE:

DIFFUSER

INHALER

TOPICAL

OTHER

MY RATING:

NOTES:

My Oil Ratings

PURPOSE OF OIL

NAME:

MY RATING:

PURPOSE OF OIL

NAME:

MY RATING:

PURPOSE OF OIL

NAME:

MY RATING:

PURPOSE OF OIL

NAME:

MY RATING:

PURPOSE OF OIL

NAME:

MY RATING:

NOTES:

My Favorite Blends

NAME:

USED FOR:

INGREDIENTS:

NOTES:

NAME:

USED FOR:

INGREDIENTS:

NOTES:

My Favorite Blends

NAME: USED FOR:

INGREDIENTS:

NOTES:

NAME: USED FOR:

INGREDIENTS:

NOTES:

Lavender Blends

DIFFUSER BLENDS

NAME: SEA BREEZE

2 DROPS LAVENDER

3 DROPS LIME

1 DROP SPEARMINT

NAME: COOL DOWN

4 DROPS SPEARMINT

2 DROPS LAVENDER

2 DROPS PEPPERMINT

NAME: PEACEFULNESS

3 DROPS LAVENDER

3 DROPS VETIVER

2 DROPS YLANG YLANG

NAME: CREATIVE SPARK

3 DROPS LAVENDER

3 DROPS SWEET ORANGE

1 DROP PEPPERMINT

NAME: OCEAN BREEZE:

4 DROPS LAVENDER

3 DROPS ROSEMARY

2 DROPS LEMONGRASS

NAME: LAVENDAR MINT

4 DROPS LAVENDER

3 DROPS PEPPERMINT

1 DROP VETIVER

NAME: CLEAN AIR

3 DROPS LAVENDER

3 DROPS TANGERINE

3 DROPS EUCALYPTUS

NAME: MINDFULNESS

2 DROPS LAVENDER

3 DROPS BERGAMOT

2 DROPS ROSEMARY

NOTES:

Wellness Blends

DIFFUSER BLENDS

NAME: ENERGIZING

4 DROPS PEPPERMINT

4 DROPS CINNAMON

2 DROPS ROSEMARY

NAME: EXTREME FOCUS

4 DROPS BALANCE

2 DROPS FRANKINCENSE

2 DROPS VETIVER

NAME: INNER CALM

3 DROPS ELEVATION

3 DROPS BERGAMOT

3 DROPS FRANKINCENSE

NAME: TRANQUILITY

3 DROPS LAVENDER

2 DROPS LIME

3 DROPS MANDARIN

NAME: LOVER OF LIFE

3 DROPS ROSEMARY

3 DROPS PEPPERMINT

3 DROPS FRANKINCENSE

NAME: STRESS BE GONE

3 DROPS LAVENDER

2 DROPS CHAMOMILE

2 DROPS YLANG YLANG

NAME: RELAXATION

3 DROPS BERGAMOT

3 DROPS PATCHOULI

3 DROPS YLANG YLANG

NAME: ACTIVE LIFE

2 DROPS GRAPEFRUIT

3 DROPS PEPPERMINT

3 DROPS ROSEMARY

NOTES:

Happiness Blends

DIFFUSER BLENDS

NAME: CHEERFUL

3 DROPS WILD ORANGE

3 DROPS FRANKINCENSE

1 DROP CINNAMON

NAME: INNER PEACE

2 DROPS PEPPERMINT

2 DROPS LAVENDER

2 DROPS WILD ORANGE

NAME: WITH PURPOSE

3 DROPS LEMON

2 DROPS OREGANO

2 DROPS ON GUARD

NAME: BOOSTER

2 DROPS LAVENDER

3 DROPS SWEET ORANGE

3 DROPS PEPPERMINT

NAME: SWEETNESS

3 DROPS BERGAMOT

2 DROPS GERANIUM

3 DROPS LAVENDER

NAME: ZONED OUT

2 DROPS ROSEMARY

2 DROPS CINNAMON

1 DROP CLOVE

NAME: LAUGHTER

3 DROPS LEMON

3 DROPS TANGERINE

2 DROPS MELALEUCA

NAME: MINDFULNESS

3 DROPS LAVENDER

3 DROPS BERGAMOT

1 DROP CLOVE

NOTES:

Well Rested Blends

DIFFUSER BLENDS

NAME: WELL RESTED

3 DROPS JUNIPER BERRY

3 DROPS CHAMOMILE

3 DROPS LAVENDER

NAME: WELL RESTED 2

4 DROPS CEDARWOOD

3 DROPS LAVENDER

1 DROP VETIVER

NAME: WELL RESTED 3

2 DROPS FRANKINCENSE

3 DROPS VETIVER

2 DROPS LAVENDER

NAME: WELL RESTED 4

3 DROPS BALANCE

2 DROPS LAVENDER

2 DROPS CHAMOMILE

NAME: WELL RESTED 5

3 DROPS LAVENDER

2 DROPS MARJORAM

2 DROPS ORANGE

NAME: WELL RESTED 6

3 DROPS LEMON

3 DROPS LAVENDER

2 DROPS PEPPERMINT

NAME: WELL RESTED 7

5 DROPS PEPPERMINT

4 DROPS EUCALYPTUS

2 DROPS MYRRH

NAME: WELL RESTED 8

3 DROPS LAVENDER

3 DROPS CHAMOMILE

1 DROP CLOVE

NOTES:

Autumn Blends

DIFFUSER BLENDS

NAME: PUMPKIN SPICE

5 DROPS CINNAMON

2 DROPS NUTMEG

3 DROPS CLOVE

NAME: SNICKERDOODLE

5 DROPS STRESS AWAY

3 DROPS CINNAMON

2 DROPS NUTMEG

NAME: FLANNEL SHEETS

5 DROPS BLACK SPRUCE

4 DROPS STRESS AWAY

4 DROPS ORANGE

NAME: SWEATER WEATHER

5 DROPS ORANGE

4 DROPS THIEVES

1 DROP GINGER

NAME: CIDER

4 DROPS ORANGE

3 DROPS CINNAMON

3 DROPS GINGER

NAME: CHANGING LEAVES

5 DROPS CLOVE

5 DROPS CEDARWOOD

5 DROPS ORANGE

NAME: GIVING THANKS

5 DROPS CINNAMON

3 DROPS ORANGE

2 DROPS NUTMEG

NAME: AUTUMN BREEZE

5 DROPS CHRISTMAS SPIRIT

2 DROPS CLOVE

1 DROP LEMON

NOTES:

Summer Blends

DIFFUSER BLENDS

NAME: SWEET SUNSHINE

3 DROPS LEMONGRASS

2 DROPS ORANGE

1 DROP PEPPERMINT

NAME: SUNNY DAYS

3 DROPS TANGERINE

3 DROPS LEMON

1 DROP PEPPERMINT

NAME: HAMMOCK TIME

2 DROPS LAVENDER

2 DROPS CEDARWOOD

2 DROPS WILD ORANGE

NAME: CITRUS TWIST

2 DROPS TANGERINE

2 DROPS GRAPEFRUIT

2 DROPS LEMON

NAME: SUMMER LOVING

2 DROPS JUNIPER BERRY

2 DROPS GRAPEFRUIT

2 DROPS WILD ORANGE

NAME: OCEAN BREEZE

3 DROPS BERGAMOT

3 DROPS LAVENDER

3 DROPS ROSEMARY

NAME: BEACH MEMORIES

2 DROPS SPEARMINT

3 DROPS TANGERINE

2 DROPS BERGAMOT

NAME: SUN KISSED

2 DROPS TEA TREE

2 DROPS LEMON

2 DROPS LIME

NOTES:

Winter Blends

DIFFUSER BLENDS

NAME: WINTER CITRUS

2 DROPS PEPPERMINT

2 DROPS LEMONGRASS

2 DROPS TANGERINE

NAME: CLASSIC WINTER

2 DROPS CEDARWOOD

2 DROPS LAVENDER

2 DROPS ROSEMARY

NAME: SNOWFLAKE

2 DROPS LAVENDER

2 DROPS LEMON

2 DROPS DIGIZE

NAME: HOLIDAY BAKING

2 DROPS CASSIA

2 DROPS VETIVER

2 DROPS LAVENDAR

NAME: SNOW DAYS

2 DROPS STRESS AWAY

2 DROPS THIEVES

2 DROPS CITRUS

NAME: COZY HOME

2 DROPS BERGAMOT

2 DROPS ORANGE

2 DROPS THIEVES

NAME: MOTHER NATURE

3 DROPS PEPPERMINT

3 DROPS LAVENDER

3 DROPS LEMON

NAME: WINTER MEMORIES

2 DROPS BERGAMOT

2 DROPS WILD ORANGE

2 DROPS EUCALYPTUS

NOTES:

Spring Blends

DIFFUSER BLENDS

NAME: WELCOME SPRING

2 DROPS GERANIUM

2 DROPS LEMON

2 DROPS GRAPEFRUIT

NAME: FRESH & CLEAN

4 DROPS GRAPEFRUIT

3 DROPS PEPPERMINT

3 DROPS CLARY SAGE

NAME: SPRING PETALS

2 DROPS YLANG YLANG

2 DROPS PEPPERMINT

2 DROPS JADE LEMON

NAME: SPRING CLEANING

2 DROPS LAVENDAR

3 DROPS LEMON

3 DROPS ROSEMARY

NAME: SPRING GARDEN

2 DROPS BASIL

2 DROPS PEPPERMINT

2 DROPS LIME

NAME: FRESH FLOWERS

5 DROPS CLARY SAGE

3 DROPS LAVENDAR

2 DROPS GERANIUM

NAME: MOTHER NATURE

3 DROPS PEPPERMINT

3 DROPS LAVENDAR

3 DROPS LEMON

NAME: GOOD MORNING

4 DROPS JOY

3 DROPS LEMON

1 DROP TANGERINE

NOTES:

Holiday Blends

DIFFUSER BLENDS

NAME: DECK THE HALLS

4 DROPS PINE

2 DROPS BLUE SPRUCE

2 DROPS CEDARWOOD

NAME: CANDY CANE

4 DROPS PEPPERMINT

3 DROPS BERGAMOT

1 DROP WILD ORANGE

NAME: SUGAR PLUM FAIRY

3 DROPS CITRUS BLISS

2 DROPS DOUGLAS FIR

2 DROPS MOTIVATE

NAME: OH, HOLY NIGHT

5 DROPS THIEVES

2 DROPS FRANKINCENSE

2 DROPS CITRUS FRESH

NAME: SNOW ANGELS

4 DROPS STRESS AWAY

3 FRESH CITRUS

1 DROP FRANKINCENSE

NAME: SPICED CIDER

3 DROPS WILD ORANGE

2 DROPS CINNAMON BARK

1 DROP CLOVE

NAME: MERRY & BRIGHT

3 DROPS LEMON

2 DROPS DOUGLAS FIR

2 DROPS CINNAMON

NAME: GINGERBREAD MAN

4 DROPS GINGER

2 DROPS CLOVES

2 DROPS CINNAMON

NOTES:

Clean House Blends

DIFFUSER BLENDS

NAME: SPARKLY CLEAN

3 DROPS LEMON

3 DROPS PEPPERMINT

3 DROPS EUCALYPTUS

NAME: NICE & TIDY

3 DROPS EUCALYPTUS

3 DROPS WILD ORANGE

3 DROPS LIME

NAME: FRESH SCENT

3 DROPS LEMON

3 DROPS EASY AIR

3 DROPS LIME

NAME: TIDY HOME

1 DROP ROSE

1 DROP CARDAMOM

2 DROPS WILD ORANGE

NAME: DECLUTTERING

4 DROPS LEMON

3 DROPS LEMONGRASS

2 DROPS PEPPERMINT

NAME: SPRING CLEANING

4 DROPS LEMON

3 DROPS LAVENDER

2 DROPS ROSEMARY

NAME: GLOSSY CLEAN

4 DROPS FRANKINCENSE

4 DROPS CYPRESS

2 DROPS YLANG YLANG

NAME: HOUSEKEEPER

2 DROPS CINNAMON

2 DROPS CARDAMOM

2 DROPS LEMOM

NOTES:

Personality Blends

DIFFUSER BLENDS

NAME: CONFIDENT

2 DROPS SPEARMINT

2 DROPS TANGERINE

2 DROPS BERGAMOT

NAME: CAREFREE

5 DROPS BERGAMOT

2 DROPS PATCHOULI

2 DROPS LIME

NAME: HAPPY

2 DROPS WILD ORANGE

2 DROPS GRAPEFRUIT

2 DROPS CLOVE

NAME: INSPIRED

1 DROP ROSE

1 DROP PURIFY

2 DROPS JUNIPER BERRY

NAME: FOCUSED

3 DROPS DOUGLAS FIR

2 DROPS LEMON

1 DROP PEPPERMINT

NAME: ENERGETIC

2 DROPS PEPPERMINT

3 DROPS GRAPEFRUIT

3 DROPS BERGAMOT

NAME: MOTIVATED

2 DROPS ELEVATION

2 DROPS CYPRESS

2 DROPS LIME

NAME: PEACEFUL

2 DROPS FRANKINCENSE

2 DROPS WHITE FIR

2 DROPS LAVENDER

NOTES:

Day to Day Blends

DIFFUSER BLENDS

NAME: SLEEP TIME

4 DROPS LAVENDER

4 DROPS CEDARWOOD

3 DROPS CHAMOMILE

NAME: ANTI-STRESS

4 DROPS BERGAMOT

4 DROPS FRANKINCENSE

1 DROP PEPPERMINT

NAME: ALLERGY BE GONE

3 DROPS LAVENDER

3 DROPS LEMON

3 DROPS PEPPERMINT

NAME: CONCENTRATION

4 DROPS LAVENDER

4 DROPS MELALEUCA

4 DROPS FRANKINCENSE

NAME: COMBAT NAUSEA

3 DROPS GINGER

5 DROPS PEPPERMINT

1 DROP BALANCE

NAME: HEADACHES

2 DROPS FRANKINCENSE

2 DROPS LAVENDER

4 DROPS PEPPERMINT

NAME: BREATHE EASY

4 DROPS PEPPERMINT

2 DROPS EUCALYPTUS

2 DROPS LEMON

NAME: IMMUNE BOOST

2 DROPS FRANKINCENSE

5 DROPS LEMON

2 DROPS PEPPERMINT

NOTES:

Essential Oil Recipes

NAME:

NAME:

NAME:

NAME:

NAME:

NAME:

NAME:

NAME:

Essential Oil Recipes

NAME:

NAME:

NAME:

NAME:

NAME:

NAME:

NAME:

NAME:

Essential Oil Wish List

NAME	USED FOR	PRICE	KID SAFE?

My Favorite Oils

ENERGY

CALMING

SLEEP

FOCUS/CLARITY

WELLNESS

ROMANCE

ANXIETY

JOYFUL

Essential Oil Inventory

NAME	USED FOR	DATE OPENED	FAVORITE?

My Favorite Blends

NAME:　　　　　　　　　　　　　　　USED FOR:

INGREDIENTS:

NOTES:

NAME:　　　　　　　　　　　　　　　USED FOR:

INGREDIENTS:

NOTES:

Essential Oil Inventory

NAME	USED FOR	DATE OPENED	FAVORITE?

Essential Oil Wish List

NAME	USED FOR	PRICE	KID SAFE?

My Favorite Oils

ENERGY

CALMING

SLEEP

FOCUS/CLARITY

WELLNESS

ROMANCE

ANXIETY

JOYFUL

Testing Out Blends

NAME:

INGREDIENTS:

PURPOSE:

DIFFUSER

INHALER

TOPICAL

OTHER

MY RATING:

NOTES:

Testing Out Blends

NAME:

INGREDIENTS:

PURPOSE:

DIFFUSER

INHALER

TOPICAL

OTHER

MY RATING:

NOTES:

Testing Out Blends

NAME:

INGREDIENTS:

PURPOSE:

DIFFUSER

INHALER

TOPICAL

OTHER

MY RATING:

NOTES:

Testing Out Blends

NAME:

PURPOSE:

INGREDIENTS:

DIFFUSER

INHALER

TOPICAL

OTHER

MY RATING:

NOTES:

My Oil Ratings

PURPOSE OF OIL

NAME:

MY RATING:

PURPOSE OF OIL

NAME:

MY RATING:

PURPOSE OF OIL

NAME:

MY RATING:

PURPOSE OF OIL

NAME:

MY RATING:

PURPOSE OF OIL

NAME:

MY RATING:

NOTES:

My Oil Ratings

PURPOSE OF OIL

NAME:

MY RATING:

PURPOSE OF OIL

NAME:

MY RATING:

PURPOSE OF OIL

NAME:

MY RATING:

PURPOSE OF OIL

NAME:

MY RATING:

PURPOSE OF OIL

NAME:

MY RATING:

NOTES:

My Oil Ratings

PURPOSE OF OIL

NAME:

MY RATING:

PURPOSE OF OIL

NAME:

MY RATING:

PURPOSE OF OIL

NAME:

MY RATING:

PURPOSE OF OIL

NAME:

MY RATING:

PURPOSE OF OIL

NAME:

MY RATING:

NOTES:

My Favorite Blends

NAME:

USED FOR:

INGREDIENTS:

NOTES:

NAME:

USED FOR:

INGREDIENTS:

NOTES:

My Favorite Blends

NAME: **USED FOR:**

INGREDIENTS:

NOTES:

....

....

....

....

NAME: **USED FOR:**

INGREDIENTS:

NOTES:

....

....

....

....

My Favorite Blends

NAME: USED FOR:

INGREDIENTS:

NOTES:

NAME: USED FOR:

INGREDIENTS:

NOTES:

My Favorite Blends

NAME:

USED FOR:

INGREDIENTS:

NOTES:

NAME:

USED FOR:

INGREDIENTS:

NOTES:

Essential Oil Inventory

NAME	USED FOR	DATE OPENED	FAVORITE?

Essential Oil Wish List

NAME	USED FOR	PRICE	KID SAFE?

My Favorite Oils

ENERGY

CALMING

SLEEP

FOCUS/CLARITY

WELLNESS

ROMANCE

ANXIETY

JOYFUL

Testing Out Blends

NAME:

INGREDIENTS:

PURPOSE:

DIFFUSER

INHALER

TOPICAL

OTHER

MY RATING:

NOTES:

My Oil Ratings

PURPOSE OF OIL

NAME:

MY RATING:

PURPOSE OF OIL

NAME:

MY RATING:

PURPOSE OF OIL

NAME:

MY RATING:

PURPOSE OF OIL

NAME:

MY RATING:

PURPOSE OF OIL

NAME:

MY RATING:

NOTES:

My Favorite Blends

NAME: USED FOR:

INGREDIENTS:

NOTES:

NAME: USED FOR:

INGREDIENTS:

NOTES:

My Favorite Blends

NAME: USED FOR:

INGREDIENTS:

NOTES:

NAME: USED FOR:

INGREDIENTS:

NOTES:

Essential Oil Inventory

NAME	USED FOR	DATE OPENED	FAVORITE?

Essential Oil Wish List

NAME	USED FOR	PRICE	KID SAFE?

My Favorite Oils

ENERGY

CALMING

SLEEP

FOCUS/CLARITY

WELLNESS

ROMANCE

ANXIETY

JOYFUL

Testing Out Blends

NAME:

PURPOSE:

INGREDIENTS:

- DIFFUSER
- INHALER
- TOPICAL
- OTHER

MY RATING:

NOTES:

My Oil Ratings

PURPOSE OF OIL

NAME:

MY RATING:

PURPOSE OF OIL

NAME:

MY RATING:

PURPOSE OF OIL

NAME:

MY RATING:

PURPOSE OF OIL

NAME:

MY RATING:

PURPOSE OF OIL

NAME:

MY RATING:

NOTES:

My Favorite Blends

NAME: USED FOR:

INGREDIENTS:

NOTES:

NAME: USED FOR:

INGREDIENTS:

NOTES:

My Favorite Blends

NAME: USED FOR:

INGREDIENTS:

NOTES:

NAME: USED FOR:

INGREDIENTS:

NOTES:

Essential Oil Inventory

NAME	USED FOR	DATE OPENED	FAVORITE?

Essential Oil Wish List

NAME	USED FOR	PRICE	KID SAFE?

My Favorite Oils

ENERGY

CALMING

SLEEP

FOCUS/CLARITY

WELLNESS

ROMANCE

ANXIETY

JOYFUL

Testing Out Blends

NAME:

INGREDIENTS:

PURPOSE:

DIFFUSER

INHALER

TOPICAL

OTHER

MY RATING:

NOTES:

My Oil Ratings

PURPOSE OF OIL

NAME:

MY RATING:

PURPOSE OF OIL

NAME:

MY RATING:

PURPOSE OF OIL

NAME:

MY RATING:

PURPOSE OF OIL

NAME:

MY RATING:

PURPOSE OF OIL

NAME:

MY RATING:

NOTES:

My Favorite Blends

NAME: USED FOR:

INGREDIENTS:

NOTES:

NAME: USED FOR:

INGREDIENTS:

NOTES:

My Favorite Blends

NAME: USED FOR:

INGREDIENTS:

NOTES:

NAME: USED FOR:

INGREDIENTS:

NOTES:

Essential Oil Inventory

NAME	USED FOR	DATE OPENED	FAVORITE?

Essential Oil Wish List

NAME	USED FOR	PRICE	KID SAFE?

My Favorite Oils

ENERGY

CALMING

SLEEP

FOCUS/CLARITY

WELLNESS

ROMANCE

ANXIETY

JOYFUL

Testing Out Blends

NAME:

INGREDIENTS:

PURPOSE:

DIFFUSER

INHALER

TOPICAL

OTHER

MY RATING:

NOTES:

My Oil Ratings

PURPOSE OF OIL

NAME:

MY RATING:

PURPOSE OF OIL

NAME:

MY RATING:

PURPOSE OF OIL

NAME:

MY RATING:

PURPOSE OF OIL

NAME:

MY RATING:

PURPOSE OF OIL

NAME:

MY RATING:

NOTES:

My Favorite Blends

NAME: USED FOR:

INGREDIENTS:

NOTES:

NAME: USED FOR:

INGREDIENTS:

NOTES:

My Favorite Blends

NAME: USED FOR:

INGREDIENTS:

NOTES:

NAME: USED FOR:

INGREDIENTS:

NOTES:

Essential Oil Inventory

NAME	USED FOR	DATE OPENED	FAVORITE?

Essential Oil Wish List

NAME	USED FOR	PRICE	KID SAFE?

My Favorite Oils

ENERGY

CALMING

SLEEP

FOCUS/CLARITY

WELLNESS

ROMANCE

ANXIETY

JOYFUL

Testing Out Blends

NAME:

INGREDIENTS:

PURPOSE:

DIFFUSER

INHALER

TOPICAL

OTHER

MY RATING:

NOTES:

My Oil Ratings

PURPOSE OF OIL

NAME:

MY RATING:

PURPOSE OF OIL

NAME:

MY RATING:

PURPOSE OF OIL

NAME:

MY RATING:

PURPOSE OF OIL

NAME:

MY RATING:

PURPOSE OF OIL

NAME:

MY RATING:

NOTES:

My Favorite Blends

NAME: USED FOR:

INGREDIENTS:

NOTES:

....

....

....

....

NAME: USED FOR:

INGREDIENTS:

NOTES:

....

....

....

....

My Favorite Blends

NAME: USED FOR:

INGREDIENTS:

NOTES:
....
....
....
....
....

NAME: USED FOR:

INGREDIENTS:

NOTES:
....
....
....
....
....

Essential Oil Inventory

NAME	USED FOR	DATE OPENED	FAVORITE?

Essential Oil Wish List

NAME	USED FOR	PRICE	KID SAFE?

My Favorite Oils

ENERGY

CALMING

SLEEP

FOCUS/CLARITY

WELLNESS

ROMANCE

ANXIETY

JOYFUL

Testing Out Blends

NAME:

PURPOSE:

INGREDIENTS:

DIFFUSER

INHALER

TOPICAL

OTHER

MY RATING:

NOTES:

My Oil Ratings

PURPOSE OF OIL

NAME:

MY RATING:

PURPOSE OF OIL

NAME:

MY RATING:

PURPOSE OF OIL

NAME:

MY RATING:

PURPOSE OF OIL

NAME:

MY RATING:

PURPOSE OF OIL

NAME:

MY RATING:

NOTES:

My Favorite Blends

NAME: USED FOR:

INGREDIENTS:

NOTES:

....
....
....
....
....

NAME: USED FOR:

INGREDIENTS:

NOTES:

....
....
....
....
....

My Favorite Blends

NAME: USED FOR:

INGREDIENTS:

NOTES:

NAME: USED FOR:

INGREDIENTS:

NOTES:

Essential Oil Inventory

NAME	USED FOR	DATE OPENED	FAVORITE?

Essential Oil Wish List

NAME	USED FOR	PRICE	KID SAFE?

My Favorite Oils

ENERGY

CALMING

SLEEP

FOCUS/CLARITY

WELLNESS

ROMANCE

ANXIETY

JOYFUL

Testing Out Blends

NAME:

INGREDIENTS:

PURPOSE:

DIFFUSER

INHALER

TOPICAL

OTHER

MY RATING:

NOTES:

My Oil Ratings

PURPOSE OF OIL

NAME:

MY RATING:

PURPOSE OF OIL

NAME:

MY RATING:

PURPOSE OF OIL

NAME:

MY RATING:

PURPOSE OF OIL

NAME:

MY RATING:

PURPOSE OF OIL

NAME:

MY RATING:

NOTES:

My Favorite Blends

NAME: USED FOR:

INGREDIENTS:

NOTES:

NAME: USED FOR:

INGREDIENTS:

NOTES:

My Favorite Blends

NAME: USED FOR:

INGREDIENTS:

NOTES:

NAME: USED FOR:

INGREDIENTS:

NOTES:

Essential Oil Inventory

NAME	USED FOR	DATE OPENED	FAVORITE?

Essential Oil Wish List

NAME	USED FOR	PRICE	KID SAFE?

My Favorite Oils

ENERGY

CALMING

SLEEP

FOCUS/CLARITY

WELLNESS

ROMANCE

ANXIETY

JOYFUL

Testing Out Blends

NAME:

INGREDIENTS:

PURPOSE:

DIFFUSER

INHALER

TOPICAL

OTHER

MY RATING:

NOTES:

My Oil Ratings

PURPOSE OF OIL

NAME:

MY RATING:

PURPOSE OF OIL

NAME:

MY RATING:

PURPOSE OF OIL

NAME:

MY RATING:

PURPOSE OF OIL

NAME:

MY RATING:

PURPOSE OF OIL

NAME:

MY RATING:

NOTES:

My Favorite Blends

NAME:　　　　　　　　　　　　　　　USED FOR:

INGREDIENTS:

NOTES:

NAME:　　　　　　　　　　　　　　　USED FOR:

INGREDIENTS:

NOTES:

My Favorite Blends

NAME:

USED FOR:

INGREDIENTS:

NOTES:

NAME:

USED FOR:

INGREDIENTS:

NOTES:

Essential Oil Inventory

NAME	USED FOR	DATE OPENED	FAVORITE?

Essential Oil Wish List

NAME	USED FOR	PRICE	KID SAFE?

My Favorite Oils

ENERGY

CALMING

SLEEP

FOCUS/CLARITY

WELLNESS

ROMANCE

ANXIETY

JOYFUL

Testing Out Blends

NAME:

INGREDIENTS:

PURPOSE:

DIFFUSER

INHALER

TOPICAL

OTHER

MY RATING:

NOTES:

My Oil Ratings

PURPOSE OF OIL

NAME:

MY RATING:

PURPOSE OF OIL

NAME:

MY RATING:

PURPOSE OF OIL

NAME:

MY RATING:

PURPOSE OF OIL

NAME:

MY RATING:

PURPOSE OF OIL

NAME:

MY RATING:

NOTES:

My Favorite Blends

NAME: USED FOR:

INGREDIENTS:

NOTES:

NAME: USED FOR:

INGREDIENTS:

NOTES:

My Favorite Blends

NAME:　　　　　　　　　　　　　　　　USED FOR:

INGREDIENTS:

NOTES:

NAME:　　　　　　　　　　　　　　　　USED FOR:

INGREDIENTS:

NOTES:

Essential Oil Inventory

NAME	USED FOR	DATE OPENED	FAVORITE?

Essential Oil Wish List

NAME	USED FOR	PRICE	KID SAFE?

My Favorite Oils

ENERGY

CALMING

SLEEP

FOCUS/CLARITY

WELLNESS

ROMANCE

ANXIETY

JOYFUL

Testing Out Blends

NAME:

INGREDIENTS:

PURPOSE:

DIFFUSER

INHALER

TOPICAL

OTHER

MY RATING:

NOTES:

My Oil Ratings

PURPOSE OF OIL

NAME:

MY RATING:

PURPOSE OF OIL

NAME:

MY RATING:

PURPOSE OF OIL

NAME:

MY RATING:

PURPOSE OF OIL

NAME:

MY RATING:

PURPOSE OF OIL

NAME:

MY RATING:

NOTES:

My Favorite Blends

NAME: USED FOR:

INGREDIENTS:

NOTES:

NAME: USED FOR:

INGREDIENTS:

NOTES:

My Favorite Blends

NAME:

USED FOR:

INGREDIENTS:

NOTES:

NAME:

USED FOR:

INGREDIENTS:

NOTES:

Essential Oil Inventory

NAME	USED FOR	DATE OPENED	FAVORITE?

Essential Oil Wish List

NAME	USED FOR	PRICE	KID SAFE?

My Favorite Oils

ENERGY

CALMING

SLEEP

FOCUS/CLARITY

WELLNESS

ROMANCE

ANXIETY

JOYFUL

Testing Out Blends

NAME:

INGREDIENTS:

PURPOSE:

DIFFUSER

INHALER

TOPICAL

OTHER

MY RATING:

NOTES:

My Oil Ratings

PURPOSE OF OIL

NAME:

MY RATING:

PURPOSE OF OIL

NAME:

MY RATING:

PURPOSE OF OIL

NAME:

MY RATING:

PURPOSE OF OIL

NAME:

MY RATING:

PURPOSE OF OIL

NAME:

MY RATING:

NOTES:

My Favorite Blends

NAME: USED FOR:

INGREDIENTS:

NOTES:

NAME: USED FOR:

INGREDIENTS:

NOTES:

My Favorite Blends

NAME: USED FOR:

INGREDIENTS:

NOTES:

NAME: USED FOR:

INGREDIENTS:

NOTES:

Essential Oil Inventory

NAME	USED FOR	DATE OPENED	FAVORITE?

Essential Oil Wish List

NAME	USED FOR	PRICE	KID SAFE?

www.ingramcontent.com/pod-product-compliance
Lightning Source LLC
Chambersburg PA
CBHW071719020426
42333CB00017B/2326